MY CATHETER AND I

MY CATHETER AND I

JOHN GIACON

Library of Congress Control Number: pending
ISBN: Hardcover   978-1-4653-5891-2
               Softcover   978-1-4653-5890-5
               Ebook   978-1-4653-5892-9

To order additional copies of this book, contact:
Xlibris Corporation
0800-891-366
www.xlibris.co.nz
Orders@Xlibris.co.nz
700209

CONTENTS

A SINCERE DEDICATION

"My Catheter and I" has been written by myself as a dedication to all members of the Auckland Hospital Board, the Doctor responsible for caring for me and for the unstinting professional services he afforded me.

Also for the care and attention I received from the many DHB Personnel—Doctors, male and female. Nurses, male and female at all hours day and night, and the various medical staff who tracked my progress for their records.

And the members of my family led by my dear wife, as well as many great friends.

I sincerely thank you all.

John Giacon

FOREWORD

Those of you who may be aware of my previous ventures into the realms of published literature will be aware that all my previous publications had a flyfishing genre. You might well ask "What on earth is John doing writing a new book with a medical background?"

In my 76th year, in fact only a week or so before my 76th birthday my journey through life was sent on a new path. And what a path it turned out to be. It was new to me and I must admit I had real problems adjusting to the twists and turns that I experienced as I progressed on this new adventure.

Before I unravel the twists and turns I have just mentioned it might help you understand the story that follows if I tell you I am New Zealander born of Italian background. I do have certain Italian traits—you know—impatience, excitability, passion, incredulity, and I can admit now to displaying all these traits plus a few others I must confess; such as temper, tantrums and anger.

To my credit though, I must inform you that amongst all my angst my good traits were always present. I could take a joke even if it was on me. I could laugh at dilemmas once I understood them, I often cried too, especially in relief when some new problem was resolved.

I really came to appreciate the support of my wife and family, I could see they wanted to help me and they did, this help was the most heartening aspect of the whole saga. I must also acknowledge the support of the medical people involved, nurses, doctors and administrators. Some were exceptionally good and I have to say some were just awful! But as this story unfolds please note that I do not use any names, to do so would be unfair and unethical.

In our country the Medical System is much maligned for things like methodology, delays, yes—mistakes as well, but let me say from personal experience that I have nothing but praise for all the personnel involved within our medical system, a cross section of whom you will meet in the following pages. I hope my story will amuse you and you will be able to laugh at my various reactions to the predicaments I found myself in.

John Giacon
The Catheter Kid

A FEW FACTS & FIGURES TO BE GOING ON WITH.

New Zealand has a population of just over four million. The female segment of our populace slightly outnumbers the male. By how many doesn't really matter because as this story unfolds you will soon discern it is of more concern to us males, yes we men are the prime targets for this missal. However, I do hope the females who read it will understand that we men do suffer from ailments afflicting parts of our anatomy, in particular our Prostate Gland. Let me welcome you to the world of Urology!

This missal in not in anyway intended to be a dissertation about the science of Urology, although let me make it clear; there is a serious science involved. No, my story is a simple account of one layman's voyage through a part of the Urology world. In fact my part in this voyage is really microscopic, however, please keep in mind it was damn well very soon of mighty Importance to me! The reason I wish to record my journey is based on the realisation that men like me somewhat ignored our meeting with Prostate during our trip through life. Were we scared about it? Were we reckless? Were we careless? Well yes, some of us were!

Back to my figures; the 450,000 male members of our population. I have been advised by some prominent medical men who should know, that 45% of men over the age of 40 will at some stage of their mature age span will require treatment related to their prostate. Stop! Think about it! That means 205,000 of us men are going to have problems.

I now have to accept as a fait accompli that I am now a prostate statistic. As I advance through my treatment of the problem I confess in the back of my mind I find myself asking if am I destined to become a fatal statistic because on this trip there have been a couple of times I felt my time had come. But thankfully, the morbid thoughts have been offset by many humorous moments and it is these moments I want to tell you about.

My style of writing has often been described as "telling it like it is", and that is my intention with this story. And throughout the tale there is one terrible underlying feature you have not yet been properly introduced to—My Catheter—in fact you will meet all 15 of them. They are an abomination, and an infliction, and yet a lifesaver. My book title has been deliberately penned as "My Catheter and I" because I want to keep my battles with all my catheters on a more or less one on one basis and to hell with using proper English! This is my book anyway.

Men who read this book and may be in a situation where they can emphasize with the facts as I present them will receive a bonus; the book would make an excellent Mother's Day present! But to male readers I urge you to make sure your sons get to read it, prepare them early, you just might improve their odds of coping with future prostate problems.

CHAPTER 1

THE RUDE AWAKENING

During the early years of my retirement I filled my spare time by writing books, and the books I wrote were about my addiction to the sport of fly-fishing. Yes, I did have an addiction and to be honest I still do, I am an avid fly-fisher and I can tell you that while some people will tell you that the next best thing to actually fly-fishing is reading about it, I found that writing about it is better still!

On reflection I now believe that those years I sat in front of my computer writing my books in a somewhat cramped position, often compressing the need to visit the toilet to have a pee for unreasonably long spells set up a condition that brought about some urgency for me to visit the toilet much more frequently than I had done normally.

I have to tell you that the frequency I had to pee became an embarrassment. Worse, I now found that I had to perform several times at night and my sleep hours were reduced considerably. Other factors had a pronounced effect on my sudden need to pee. For example the sound of running water when I turned on the tap made me literally run for the nearest toilet. I had become a bloody fountain! On a few occasions I simply struggled to hang on and some leaking occurred. Let me ask now—has this happened to you? Yet?

It became so bad I visited my Doctor who subscribed some pills to help alleviate the situation. He told me the problem emanated from my prostate gland and that sooner or later I would have to face an operation to put things right. Every time I went to my Doctor from then on he never failed to inquire how I was managing my peeing control and he never forgot to mention the need to have an operation. I recall asking him what such an operation involved and he explained it to me. I asked him what the cost might be and he nonchalantly told me about $3000.

I put up with the inconvenience for a couple of years and in fact whenever I was going anywhere, be it a long drive or a visit to friends or family, I established a mental picture of where convenient toilets were located in case of peeing emergencies. That is when it dawned on me why toilets were also called conveniences; funny that, isn't it?

It was in April 2011 and my 76th birthday was approaching when my peeing urges stopped—completely! While I still felt the need to pass water I just couldn't! I hadn't been able to pee no matter how I tried. I went 23 hours without a drop, so somewhat in a panic I went back to my Doctor. He showed some impatience and said he was fed up with my lack of willingness to take some positive action.

There and then he picked up his telephone and made me an appointment to visit a Urology Specialist the very next day.

When I arrived at the specialist's rooms, which were in the five star class; I met his receptionist who greeted me by asking if my bladder was full? As I hadn't passed water for a very long time I told her I supposed it was. She took me to a fancy toilet especially designed to collect my contribution and analyse it ready for the Specialist. Would you believe it? I couldn't perform! Nothing at all.

The unflappable receptionist made me drink eight glasses of water and then back to the toilet to try again. Still nothing. She advised the Specialist who decided to see me anyway and expressed the hope that I could oblige before I left. My examination was about to begin. This was the key moment my life pattern was about to be changed.

Why is it that when you have a prostate examination the examiner dons little white gloves and enters you body via your rectum? I knew what was coming as over past years I had been subjected to similar inspections. Nevertheless the procedure sends me virtually clawing at the wall as I try to escape the indignity. To make the situation worse, the Specialist exclaimed—"My God, this must be the biggest prostate I have ever come across!" How do you think I felt?

To make matters worse he said to me while I was still recovering on the couch "You definitely need an operation, we may have to cut you open! Such an operation will cost $20,000!"

I replied, "You're joking, I can't afford that" as I recalled my Doctor telling me an operation would cost $3000. Believe me I had just experienced a really rude awakening. I felt like asking if there was a heart specialist in the building.

I could tell by the curtailing of any small talk or normal pleasantries that any professional interest in my case had gone out the window. I wasn't even asked to try to pass water again. The receptionist handed me an invoice for $390, which my wife paid for; and it was a case of there is the door good bye. But the very next morning the receptionist phoned me and advised that if I did decide to proceed there was a Cardiology test required and that would cost an additional $6000. I said, "Forget it" and hung up. I probably did need a heart examination by then!

Obviously the professional medical people had assumed I carried medical insurance to cover such exorbitant costs, but the fact is that on attaining the age of 70 my wife and I decided that having to pay in excess of $5500 each for cover was just more than we could afford, so we cancelled our insurance.

So that is the opening chapter to what I believe started me and my dear wife out on a new adventure full of as many twists and turns that you might find in a Catheter as certainly happened to me.

CHAPTER 2

TO PEE OR NOT TO PEE

I now found myself in quite a dilemma. Following my visit to the Specialist I was still not able to urinate properly. Over the next few days I would occasionally pee like the proverbial fountain and experience a great sense of relief, although to be honest I did need to strain my bladder to make it happen, and there was some pain involved. But alas, despite my straining, more often than not nothing happened, not even a trickle, yet there were different degrees of pain.

Obviously I couldn't carry on under these circumstances, so it was back to my Doctor. Once again he didn't stuff around—"I am sending you to the Emergency Clinic at Auckland Hospital" he said, "I will fax them ahead of you asking that they make a serious examination of you and suggest they insert a Catheter as an interim measure pending an operation".

So it was off to Auckland Hospital, and because I didn't have a clue what was going to happen to me I got my wife to drive me there where I was duly admitted. I was registered as a patient and taken to a small room and asked to wait until a nurse came to see me.

About an hour later the nurse arrived and I can tell you that the waiting time was not wasted, at least five times I followed my urge to pee and visited the adjacent toilet, but nothing was forthcoming. The young nurse was most pleasant and efficient. In a matter of minutes she had checked my blood pressure, taken a blood sample, pricked my finger to check my blood sugar level, stuck some new fangled type of thermometer in my ear to read my temperature.

Once the nurse had completed gathering my statistics she told us these would be collated and presented to whichever Doctor would be handling my case and he would be along shortly. Another hour passed with me lying prostrate on the bed with my poor wife reading a magazine and urging me to be patient and stay calm. It was very hard to take her advice; I was very frustrated. 'All good things come to those who wait' is a platitude I find hard to accept, but I had no choice did I?

My Doctor duly arrived and in accordance with my earlier advice he shall like all medical personnel in this narrative will remain nameless. Suffice to say he was Chinese, young and very pleasant and most polite. Now it was a case of stripping off my lower clothing and finding myself being prodded and poked in full view of the nurse and my wife, who of course was probably bored having seen it all before. I have to admit I was nevertheless somewhat embarrassed.

At the conclusion of his examination the Hospital Doctor said he agreed with my personal doctor's recommendation that pending a possible operation I should be fitted with a Catheter to relieve my peeing problem and that he would proceed forthwith. Various trolleys were wheeled into the room with all manner of instruments and plastic covered packets that make up the Catheter segments. This was the moment My Catheter and I were going to be introduced to each other. It proved to be an unforgettable moment.

Forgive me if I take some trouble to describe what happened next. The poking and prodding continued. The Catheter insertion of the tube into my penis was hardly exquisite. As he made the initial insertion my Chinese doctor kept saying 'sorry—sorry'. I am sure the involuntary grimacing and clenching of teeth and my frequent beseeches to God were give away signs of my extreme discomfort. I tried not to writhe about on the bed. I looked to my wife seeking some kind of solace, but all she did was give me a radiant smile back. Perhaps she considered this was 'pay back' time for any pain I had caused her!

My Chinese doctor completed his part of the fitting and asked the nurse to clean me up and fit a leg bag to the drainage section of the Catheter. My Catheter and I now had both an internal and external connection, but I can tell you now this connection never became an amicable relationship as you will learn, it was the beginning a loathing and I do believe it was a mutual feeling.

The doctor returned shortly to check the catheter was doing its job and advised me he would register me to attend a forthcoming Urology Clinic at Green Lane Hospital in about four weeks time. I was then discharged four hours after my admission and on my discharge paper I was described as having a second episode of acute urine retention most likely due to BHP. He has failed TROC in the community and came for IDC insertion. Please don't ask me what all the Capital Letters mean, I just don't know.

So I left the hospital supposedly a new man. I knew I was walking somewhat strangely due to parts of my attached tubing not seeming to follow my general direction. I was sure people would notice my hesitant action and wonder what the matter was with me. I was self—conscious, I was certainly aware I was carrying a catheter, there were new sensations emanating from it, things like a pressure on the eye of my penis. I was well aware that the catheter was doing its job, the appearance of fluid in the leg bag was ample evidence that I had peed and there was no real pain whatsoever.

Apart from the mental anxiety due to my catheters presence in my anatomy and the extreme annoyance it caused me when I sensed and resented it's presence when I was moving about, and especially when I went to bed at night and was losing many hours of sleep, I have to admit that I suffered hardly any pain whatsoever, in fact I felt fine. As I found at it was the 'lull before the storm!'

Only two days after my catheter insertion I received a phone call from the District Nursing Service that they had been advised of my visit to Auckland Hospital and I could expect a visit by their nurses in two days time to follow up the work done by the Hospital staff. The main purpose of the visit was to remove the catheter to see if my peeing had returned to normal. They would return after four hours and if things had returned to normal that would mean goodbye to my catheter. I was ecstatic.

So early on the fourth day two young nurses arrived and it was time to disrobe and let them do their thing. My Catheter and I parted company with very little trouble; in fact the pain was minimal. They cleaned up the remainder of their items and said they would be back later. Over those four hours 'Too Pee or not Pee' became the project for the day. I had the urge the whole time and I tried and tried, but you guessed it, nothing happened!

The lovely District Nurses seemed to genuinely regret explaining to me that as I hadn't performed they would have to insert a new catheter! I was crestfallen, but I had to do what I was told. It seemed to me that all I had undergone prior to this new invasion of my body had been a waste of time. I agreed to the nurses doing their thing.

So once again I had to undergo the special pains of having a tube pushed up my penis. Only this time the experience was far more prolonged, in fact unbelievably, as I lay there, making groaning noises and listening to repeated 'sorry—sorry' exclamations I sensed something was wrong.

My concerns that something wasn't going to plan was confirmed when the senior nurse said to her accomplice in a whisper, "we have a tricky dickey here". Despite the predicament I found myself in I burst out laughing much to the embarrassment of the two nurses. But hell's bells, it was really funny and it endeared me to the two young women who were trying to help me.

The upshot of the nurse's efforts was they had to tell me they couldn't manage to fit a second catheter and I should contact my doctor for advice. My doctor was not amused even when I repeated the tricky dickey episode to him. He ordered me to revisit the Emergency ward at the AHB and he would phone ahead and let them know I was coming. I could tell I was now well into the System.

CHAPTER 3

HERE WE GO AGAIN—WHOOPEE.

My Catheter experiences now entered another phase. On admittance into the Emergency Ward I was put through the same pre fitting tests as on my first visit. A young nurse checked my blood pressure, my blood sugar levels, took blood, recorded my temperature and this time used a what she called a 'Tummy Scanner' machine to record the fluid levels I was holding in my abdomen.

The Doctor arrived about an hour later and I was pleased to renew acquaintance with my Chinese doctor who attended me on my first visit. He was curious as to what had happened to the first catheter he had inserted so I had to tell him the whole story as I related to you in the previous chapter, including the 'tricky dickey' comment.

"What do they mean by tricky dickey?" asked the doctor, and upon realisation of the meaning behind the comment he burst out laughing and said to the nurse who was also laughing " there's nothing tricky about this old dickey is there nurse?" I had to join in the laughter, even though it was my 'old fella' they were laughing about. Bloody hell, this dickey had been a lifelong working tool and had served me well!

The doctor said he would insert Catheter two shortly, and instructed the still blushing young nurse to wheel in the paraphernalia he would need to do the job. So I lay on the bed exposed from waste down waiting for something to happen. I must have been there for another hour but I was patient, if you find yourself in this kind of situation you need to realise the doctors and nurses must also attend to other cases and other supportive medical staff are all in a hustle and bustle as cases are attended to.

As I lay there waiting I was surprised at the number of new faces that came into my room, hesitated a moment before apologising and hastily retreating, mostly female nurses. Then the penny dropped! Perhaps word about the 'tricky dickey' had spread around the ward and these unexpected visitors wanted to see for themselves! Maybe the 'old fella' was now a candidate for some late lifetime fame! Anyway I found a bed towel and covered up the object on show. I was possibly now classed as a spoilsport.

Do you know that as I paused in my writing a whole new thought came to me? It was like a bombshell! There is a strong possibility that the District Nurses term "a tricky dickey" is a plain and simple term of reference related to a specific problem they may come across during their work! Of course! Plain logic suggests that it is a damned good term at that. I will definitely ask the next District Nurse who comes to attend to my needs if I am thinking correctly. And in any case, if it is not their term of reference already they are welcome to it. I don't have any claim to the term because I did in fact hear it from a District Nurse in the first place. I hope that before you reach the end of this missal I will have an answer for you.

Back came my doctor who expertly inserted my catheter No 2 and checked all was in working order before discharging me. He did say he had some good news in that he had booked me into the Green Lane Hospital Urology Clin1c and that they would send me dates and time in due course. So five hours after admission I was discharged. On reflection I reckoned that of those five hours two AHB personnel, the doctor and nurse were directly attending me upon. But thinking a bit deeper into the time, it is not hard to realise that behind the scenes there must be more medical people involved. Just the administration factor must require hours as well. Don't knock our medical system; it is top class.

It took less than two days for my catheter No 3 to object to being placed in my body. No 3 went on strike! I awoke in the middle of the night with painful sensations in my abdomen. I inspected No 3 leg bag and it was dry, no fluid whatsoever! And yet I had this strong urge to pee and I just couldn't. I knew something was wrong so I dressed myself and told my wife I was going back to the hospital, and off I went at 4 am in the morning!

My admission sheet records that I arrived at 4 am and the preliminary examination revealed acute urinary retention and pain. I was diagnosed as having a blocked IDC and this was my third catheter problem. Once again I was half undressed and laid out on the bed. Once again the nurse undertook all the preliminary checks I have previously described and once again it became a waiting game.

I lay there for five hours and during that time several medical staff visited me. I listened in as they expressed opinions to each other and a consensus seemed to be emerging that besides a possible blockage in my catheter tubes I might also have a hydration problem.

I still cant believe I had a hydration problem because ever since the urine retention appeared I had religiously drank litres of water every day; I even considered adding water to my whisky as an extra measure but alas I did not have any whisky in the house. Drinking litres of water each day is one of the Cardinal rules of Urology practise, and the medical staff involved keeps insisting you drank your quota. The 'drinking water ritual' became even more important as I progressed through my prostate treatment further down the line.

About mid day two doctors arrived in my room and the principal doctor was an ebullient Scottish lady who got into her work straight away. She told me that she was going to change the type of catheter from a 16 Fr to an 18 Fr 3 way. The new type had two attachments to the main tube; these attachments provided scope for clearing blockages and flushing out.

Then she proceeded with the insertion of My Catheter No 4 with the help of the junior doctor and a nurse. I could tell by the deference the two juniors paid to the Scotch lassies commands and demands that here was a lady who was an expert and commanded respect. Once the new insertion was completed there were some tests done via the flushing out and the doctor said she was satisfied with the job. She said there should be no further problems with catheters, but if there was any more blocking to come back to the ED immediately.

I was greatly impressed by this lassies attitude and skill, particularly in the way she did her work and made sure her helpers did theirs and knew what it was all about. As she made her farewells I complimented her on her style and made a genuine comment that I felt she would be a doer and leader in any field she ventured into. I was certainly most impressed.

After a couple of more tests by the nurse I was finally discharged, nearly 12 hours after I had been admitted. I headed this chapter "Here we go again WHOO**PEE**" with emphasis on the PEE. On leaving the hospital I had a sense that now something special would happen, I was on a new road. It did happen—Alas!

CHAPTER 4.

NOT A HAPPEE CHAPPEE!

Author's note: Before continuing with my missal, let me tell you that further to the 'tricky dickey' episode in the previous chapter, today I had a visit by a District Nurse. I wont tell you the reason for the visit just yet as there are a few chapters to go before all is revealed. But I can tell you at this point that during her administrations I did interrupt her to ask if the term 'tricky dickey' was possibly a professionally used expression by members of her trade. She was adamant that it wasn't; or at least; she never used it. I apologised for asking as I may have offended her. Now I am in a quandary—should I ask another nurse? I will let you know if I do.

Only two days after receiving My Catheter 4 I was in trouble again, No 4 was like its predecessor just not performing! My admittance paper described me as a 75-year-old man discharged the previous Saturday (9th April) returning with acute urinary retention—blocked IDC—3x episodes. Patient represented with no urine output for 15 hours with 3 way IDC in situ. This was his third presentation in the week. He is awaiting urology outpatient clinic. Flushed by nurse with 500 ml, no haematuria.

PVC Bladder scan showed no urine in bladder.
Impression—no urine output and ARF due to dehydration rather than blockage.
Given IVF and draining urine well and remained comfortable.

I had driven myself to the hospital and was admitted at 02.57 in the morning and discharged at 14.32. I was there for more that 11 hours! No wonder I was not a happy chappy. There were some saving factors however. For this visit my doctor had an outgoing personality and a great sounding baritone voice. I asked him in Italian if he was of Italian origin, and he replied no he was Russian, and went on his way having a good chuckle as he wished me all the best.

The nurse attended to me for the next few hours—spasmodically. Now and then she would check the No 5 catheter was performing which it was. She did another flushing and then left me alone connected to a large drainage bag, which lay on the floor next to my bed. It lay there for another two hours until she returned to make sure it was working. She commented that her superiors were discussing if I should be shifted upstairs into a ward.

I was left waiting for another hour before she returned and told me I could go home now! I was quite flabbergasted! There was I lying half naked on the bed attached to a large catheter bag that was half full of fluid which I didn't know what to do with or how to deal with. To make matters worse she just walked away and left me there! I was quite indignant; I lay there on the bed for another half hour until I was able to attract the attention of a passing nurse and was able to ask her to find out for me just what was happening.

My original nurse returned and in total silence changed my bag to a leg bag, handed me a large brown paper bag which contained my personal items and left me to get dressed and find my way out to the discharge area where I was handed my discharge papers. That nurse, and I do know her name, was probably the one nurse in all of this experience let herself and her team down.

Also in early April I received an official letter from the Auckland DHB Eligibility Team to determine if I qualified for the right to publicly funded health care and was therefore eligible to receive free or subsidised health and disability services. The letter contained a list of the various items I needed to provide to prove I was eligible and I was happy to procure and forward them copies as requested.

Do you know I soon discovered some anomalies in my official papers that might have led to questions being asked? My Birth certificate carried the name Giovanni Battista Giacon and as I had supplied that certificate in applying for my passport it too carried the name Giovanni Giacon.

Fortunately I had some years prior to this request had an affidavit added to my passport stating that I was commonly known as John Giacon.

That did the trick and I was accepted. I then realised that with acceptance I was now going to have part of my Social Security tax payments over 59 years utilised for health reasons. I was getting some benefit for being honest over all those years, most of my lifetime in fact. Yi**PEE!**

I awoke from a good nights sleep on the 17/04/11, which was three days before my 76th birthday and was dismayed to find Catheter No 5 had failed to perform; the bag was empty. No stuffing about as my personal doctor would have said, I drove myself back to hospital and was admitted at 7.15 am. This time I had come prepared for the usual long waits and just as well I did. I grabbed one of my fly fishing books—'The Magic Hour' to read while I waited.

Once again I was submitted to all the preliminary checks, the whole nine yards as it were. My doctor for this visit was very young man and a kiwi. Under his instructions a nurse scanned my stomach and determined that I was holding 600 mls of fluid which she proceeded to drain out. The 3 Way catheter I was fitted with greatly aided the proceeds. It was determined that the poor flow was partly due to blood clots being present. These were flushed away and the doctor fitted another Catheter—No 6 that was also a 3 Way model.

Just prior to being discharged the young doctor called in to say his farewells when he observed my Magic Hour fly fishing book on the bedside table. He asked me if I was interested in fly-fishing to which I replied yes and he picked up the book to have a closer look at it and exclaimed, "You wrote this book?" which I affirmed. "I am a fly fisher also", he declared, "albeit a new one". Instantly the "Brotherhood of the Angle" became a part of our relationship. This 'Brotherhood' is renowned worldwide. I asked him to take the book which he did readily shaking my hand enthusiastically. He promised to let me have his opinion somewhere down the line.

I was discharged at 12.15 pm, but do you know the time had just flown. All the time he was in attendance on me we talked about our sport, perhaps in the future I should request fly fishers to attend upon me.

CHAPTER 5

PRESS ON REGARDLESS.

My catheter problems were persisting, it was now into May and I was becoming quite downhearted. Actually the No 6 catheter was performing well and I was able to live with it reasonably well. But then I developed an irritating itch right in the urethra opening that seemed to be growing stronger. It wasn't painful at all, just annoying, as I was conscious of it all the time.

When the District Nurse made her visit I told her about it so she had a look and advised me to visit my doctor which I did the same day. My doctor also had a look, had his nurse take a blood and urine sample and prescribed some anti biotic pills for me to take. I procured the pills from my Chemist on the way home and started taking then right away.

The itch subsided so to my way of thinking the pills were doing the job. I was very much surprised when on the Monday morning the doctor contacted me and told me to stop taking the pills immediately as the test results from the laboratory showed I apparently had an elegy towards them. Naturally I did as I was told, but the itch had gone anyway.

About this time I was working at my computer when I decided to learn more about Catheters and Urology. Yes, it's another look at facts and figures. So it was into Google and I dialled up Catheters. I was astounded to see that I could gain reference to nine and a half million descriptions! There were even pages I could visit on Trade Me. I should have hung on to my discarded catheters; I may have made a few dollars on the side! Anyone like a second hand catheter?

Seriously, there are a great many catheters covering a huge range of applications, both male and female. There are innumerable drawings of different designs and I was tempted to include a couple in this missal, but of course to do so might be interpreted as plagiarism so I will avoid the temptation.

I next dialled up Urology and again the result was staggering! I could gain reference to 55,600,000 items of Urology. Really! Hey, again there are pages of Urology based items on Ebay. But if you wanted to you could circumnavigate the world several times visiting hundreds of Urology departments, practitioners, associates, and obtain innumerable publications. I reckon a University Student could write a splendid thesis on the subject of urology working solely off the Google information. As I said—'staggering'—take a look for yourself some time.

The next exciting happening was a letter from the Urology Clinic at Green Lane Hospital summoning me to attend a clinic session on the 4th of May. The letter provided me with a list of items they wanted me bring to the clinic. The letter was exciting to me because it meant new progress was being made.

On arrival I was duly registered and had to once again undergo a gamut of tests. There were the tests I had now experienced several times, the blood pressure, blood sugar, blood tests, even my weight and height. I had to sit with a clinician and discuss my list of pills, which was quite lengthy. They wanted to know the reasons for taking some of the pills and I truthfully answered them.

When I had completed the preliminaries to their satisfaction I was next ushered into the office of the man who would decide my fate—my Surgeon. In keeping with my 'No names—no pack drill' policy from this point onwards I will only refer to him as: My Surgeon".

The Surgeon spent some time asking me questions related to why I had sought medical attention. I told him that all I really wanted was to pee comfortably! He then told me to drop my lower clothes, hop up on the bed and face the wall. I immediately knew I was in for the old "Hands on" inspection, or should I say hand in? My inspection by rectum was completed and I was told to dress and sit down.

The Surgeon then told me I had an exceptionally enlarged prostate and he had no hesitation in recommending an operation. I asked him "what does that mean?" and he blandly replied "That means you are now in the system, you are now a registered Urology patient and will be operated on in due course". I next asked when that was liable to be and all he said was "In about four weeks, you will be advised by mail". He then handed me a prescription for a drug that helps to shrink the prostate. I noticed the prescription was for an eight-week supply!

Well it now became a matter of waiting for the notice to arrive, but in the meantime my current catheter decided to intervene again. One morning I discovered I had wet myself during the night. I took myself to the bathroom to inspect the damage and lo and behold I passed urine again. But not into my catheter bag but directly out one of the small attachments to the main tube. The urine was bypassing the drainage tube.

What the bloody hell could I do? I decided it was back to the Hospital again and had myself admitted. I was promptly attended to by a nurse who obviously didn't want me peeing around the place so she said she would summon doctor post haste. I jokingly asked her if there were any fly-fishing doctors on duty and she said she would check for me.

Lo and behold, my young fly fishing doctor showed up. He quickly determined that there was a spigot missing from one of the main tube attachments. A type of plastic cork is the best way to describe it. He fossicked about in the adjacent cupboards and produced the stopper and fitted it to the attachment. The leak was successfully bunged up, but I must say that the stopper was quite large and it now became an additional irritant I could attribute to my catheter hanging about there amongst the family jewels!

My fly fisher doctor and I were able to have quite a good chat about our sport, we discussed things like favoured locations, favourite flies, the gear we used, catches we had made, a broad range of things fly fishers just love to talk about. The upshot of this second meeting was that I undertook to mail him a few more of my books, which I did.

I was in the process of leaving the building when I heard my name being paged on the hospital loudspeaker system, so I returned and there was my flyfisher doctor waiting for me. He told me that he had discussed my case with his supervisor and they had decided it might be prudent to remove my current catheter and replace it with a new one. So it was back into my room where in only a matter of minutes it was out with the old and in with n new. I left the hospital wearing Catheter No 7! I don't know why, but I was quite pleased with myself. I felt like I was someone special.

CHAPTER 6

DO WHAT YOU ARE TOLD
AND YOU'LL BE OK.

The Pre Operation Clinic I attended at Green Lane Hospital was in a way a softening up process, which was an effective way to get you ready for what was coming. You did meet up with your surgeon who gave you a cursory explanation of what was going to happen to you. Next you met your anaesthetist who discussed with you just what his role would be at your operation. He also asked a host of questions which he explained were designed to make sure you were fit enough to face the complexities involved in the forthcoming operation.

There was a very efficient nurse who took you from meeting one of the key persons in your visit to hospital to the next. In a way she was the go—between who made the whole visit function smoothly. At the conclusion of my visit she handed me a small four-page instruction pamphlet to take home to read carefully in preparation for the day of my operation. I have to say the little booklet was concise and a great help. I must have read it and re-read it many times. I was well prepared.

I was also given two other small booklets. The first carried the title **YOUR ANAESTHETIC** and again was a precise document. It carried full information on the various aspects of anaesthetics before and after application. If you had any concerns on how anaesthetics will or might affect you then here again was a very reassuring booklet. Let's face it, there can be complications and there are risk factors. Anaesthetists are probably the most intensely trained professionals in the Medical world. I presume and hope anyone having an operation involving anaesthetic receives a copy of this booklet.

The second booklet was a nine-page publication titled **TRANSURETHRAL RESECTION OF THE PROSTATE (TURP)** Patient information. Here is a really concise publication explaining the whole saga of prostate awareness from causes, complications, treatment, remedies, operations, recovery; including Pelvic Muscle Training. Let me take this opportunity to urge all men to go out of their way to obtain a copy of the TURP booklet, apply to the local District Health Board or ask your doctor to get a copy for you.

Ladies, in the beginning of this missal I suggested to male readers that they could pass a copy of this book onto their partners as a Mothers Day gift. Certainly I was being a bit facetious, but please believe me, the TURP book would really make a great gift for Fathers Day!

The last document I received was a one-page publication titled **ORDA** (Operating Room Direct Admissions). I had been advised that my reporting time into the Auckland Hospital was June 10th at 7.10 am—which I duly did. I was escorted into the Orda Room where my details were recorded and an ID bracelet attached to my wrist. I was then shown around the room by the charge nurse who then asked me several routine questions to complete her checklist and took my blood pressure, pulse and temperature.

Next I was taken to a side room where I had a very long session with my anaesthetist. He again asked me a lot of questions and then told me he still had to decide just what method of administrating anaesthetic would be used for my operation, he and my surgeon would decide shortly. Obviously here was a case of doing what I was told. I really had no choice did I?

Then, I was shown into another room to meet with my surgeon, where he explained to me that there were three options they had to select from before they would operate. One was to use a tube via my uthera to reduce the prostate, or they would cut me open and operate direct on the prostate, or they could remove the prostate entirely via the cut. He intended to make an internal inspection first using a microscopic camera. My surgeon smiled at me, shook my hand and assured me he knew what he was doing. Again I didn't really have a choice did I?

So the nurse then placed me on a wheeled cot which was to become my operating table and I was taken into a large room where there were several other similar cots waiting. I guessed this was a pre-op room and probably a recovery room also. Anyway, I was given an injection and some kind of object was fitted into my arm by my elbow. I remember being trundled into another room at about 9.30 am. I suppose this was my operating room. I can't tell you anything more because I can't recall what happened next.

I came to still on the cot as I was being wheeled into a wardroom on the 7th floor. It was 1.10 pm. I was transferred onto a bed and gradually became aware that I now had some kind of intravenous drip feed bag suspended from a bed frame dripping into the arm aperture that had been prepared before the operation. I also had an oxygen supply being pumped through each of my nostrils. At the foot of my bed there were two suspended bags feeding water into my uthera. I became aware that I had been fitted with yet another catheter (No 8), which was discharging bloody fluid into a large bag lying on the floor.

I was drowsy and dozing off for short periods, but I was very comfortable and did not have any residual pain at all. There were regular visits and inspections by the ward nurses about every 30 minutes. They checked all the various bag attachments, my oxygen supply, and my catheter No 8, all of which were performing ok. Mid afternoon they propped me up higher in my bed and I was able to observe that there were four other patients in the ward. I gave a feeble wave to the guys opposite me and one of them waved back; we gave each other a smile

About 4 pm a trio of doctors including my surgeon paid a visit. My surgeon told me it had been a major operation and I was now carrying quite a sizeable internal wound. I would have to wear the catheter for a couple of days at least until things settled down and possibly for a few days after I was discharged, however he was confident I would recover well and be back to normal in a short time.

I have tried to describe my hospital entry and operation procedures in a sort of matter of fact style because to be honest it all happened in a matter of fact kind of way. It really was a case of doing what you were told and you would be ok. But I am about to move into the next phase of My Catheter and I adventures or should I say misadventures.

At this moment in time as I wrote this chapter, I have to tell you that three full months since I first started out on this now epic trip I was still trying and waiting to have a proper pee!

CHAPTER 7.

YIPEE—THE ROAD TO RECOVERY.

Saturday the 11th of June, the morning after my operation day. I had slept on and off during my first night in the Ward and I welcomed breakfast when it arrived, at least I was hungry. I met nurses who had been on night duty and they told me everything was functioning as expected. I was vaguely conscious of staff nurses coming and going during the night as they checked the equipment dripping stuff into me and draining it out. I also met nurses coming on duty for the day shift.

At this stage in my story it is appropriate that I mention the nursing staff, male and female. I found them a caring group of people dedicated to their patient's health and welfare. Much of their work is 'hands on' and you could feel their professional skill as they administered to your needs. Being looked after by a smiling and solicitous person is reassuring and it is curative. I can only commend them to you.

The doctors made their early morning rounds visiting the patients they had operated on. My Surgeon told me, and his colleagues I had received a major operation, the average prostate is around 35 mm, mine was 204 mm, however all had gone smoothly and he expected a speedy recovery.

The rest of the day was spent simply dozing off and being awakened when our nursing staff did their thing, and by visitors coming in to see their family or friends. My ward mates were Bob, Khan and Trevor, prostate problems had brought us together and three of us were wearing catheters while the fourth had a more complicated type of catheter due to having suffered a more complicated prostate problem.

Trevor who was an aviator told us the dozing off we were experiencing was termed "zoning sleep" by aircraft crew. He said pilots and crew did it frequently when flying their aircraft and it was really quite safe. Oh yeah thought I, now pull the other one, but when he explained the logic in using zones for sleep as long as some crew members were awake it seemed reasonable to me.

Rob who had been operated on the day before us others was already up and walking about. He was fitted with a hip catheter, which travelled about with him. He was able to shower on his own and pay visits to other patients on floor seven of the ward. The other three of us were still confined to our beds, where we were body washed by a young strong male nurse. We three envied Bob his freedom.

That afternoon when our visitors had been and gone we took the opportunity to tell each other about ourselves, our livelihoods, families and exchange pleasantries to pass the time away. Except Khan who didn't appear to want to talk much at all, he just remained in his sleep zone.

But that evening after dinner had been delivered and tea or coffee served, a new batch of visitors came and went, except in Khan's case. He had visitors coming in continuously, at one stage there were 30 people crowded around his bed all talking in loud Hindi dialects, and all laughing and jabbering away happily. At this stage I began to think that perhaps Khan was a swami or Hindi monk of repute. Perhaps he was a Maharajah with his followers coming to pay homage to him. By the way, these people brought with them all manner of sweetmeats and food items. It was party time.

Things quietened down about 9.30 pm with most of Khan's guests having departed. But it didn't end there. Khan followed up his celebratory evening carry on by bringing out two or three cell phones and making contact with people all around the country and holding two or three way conversations, all in the high pitched tones and all in Hindi. Around 11 pm both Bob and I had had enough. We both made throat-clearing noises and Khan must have got the message, he put the phones away.

We were just drifting off into sleep when suddenly Khan burst into an amazing bout of snoring! I have never heard such snoring in my life! It was a veritable cacophony and I believe it was in Hindi as well! Thankfully a night nurse came to the rescue and turned the snoring champion of the world on his side.

There was yet another aspect of sharing a hospital ward I was able to experience. I can only describe it as a Dawn Chorus! As patients began to stir there was gentle coughing graded up to some quite raucous coughing? Mixed up with the coughs were many bursts of farting; again the farts ranged from gentle to raucous, and in fact I believe the louder coughs were deliberate attempts to disguise the louder farts. I have to confess I even joined in and it was widespread over the whole 7th floor. Disgusting you might say, but it was actually funny and delightful.

Sunday was an eventful day. After breakfast we were again visited by a troupe of doctors and I was told today my catheter would be removed and if I was able to pass urine freely I would be able to go home. It was bloody marvellous, the catheter was gone and I could move about freely. I was able to shower and what a great feeling that was.

So in our part of the ward we four were now armed with small receptacles to pee into and if we passed more than 120 ml we could be discharged. One by one my mates made the grade. Trevor was first, mid morning he came out of the toilet and showed the nurse on duty his results and was most pleased to be allowed to go home. We made our farewells and continued on with our own efforts. Next was Rob and he was pleased to contact his family and request they come to pick him up.

Khan and I failed the test so we were told we had to remain for another night. I was quite disconsolate. I had tried mightily to no avail, despite trying 20 or more times I could not produce more than five mls. Hells bells, I was no better off than when this journey had begun, probably worse off. To worsen my disposition, another catheter was inserted to see me through the night. Ironically catheter No 9 worked well.

That night the Hindi Festival continued, again about 30 people visited Khan and there was standing room only around our beds. My wife and daughter visited me and found it hard to converse over the din. During the day I had only had Khan for company and discovered he was a Fiji born Indian, a Hindi yes, but with no special rank at all, he was a warehouse worker in Auckland. In fact he didn't know half the people who visited him, to them it was a social occasion. To me it was a local version of Bollywood!

I had a really bad night, and yet I have to say Khan behaved himself well, no cell phones and no snoring. I was plain and simple disheartened and mentally in something of turmoil—what was wrong? Would I ever come right?

CHAPTER 8

NON-DESPERADO

I have selected the "Don't Despair" heading for this chapter as it unfolds my stay in hospital after my June 10th operation. I have already described the traumas of our first recovery day, which saw two of our roommates discharged while my Hindi mate and I didn't make the grade, which involved passing enough urine into a receptacle to earn a discharge. The doctors morning visit was merely a formality, in effect we were told pee or else!

Both Khan and I did try several times and in mid afternoon a jubilant cry from Khan announced he had made it! He was discharged and I was now the sole survivor of our little band. I tried even harder but could still only produce dribbles. This was when my feeling of despair started to set in. I tried standing in front of the bathroom basin with the tap running while I stared into the mirror saying prayers to all the saints whose names I could remember. Still not enough and I was morose and very concerned.

Late afternoon the team of doctors were again doing their rounds of the ward and when they came to me they debated whether to reinsert a catheter or leave me without one for the night in the hope I might be successful. They chose to leave me and I was and told to make sure I kept the night nurses aware of any progress. All the time I was getting urges to pass urine and I would get out of bed and visit the bathroom, but to no avail. I told myself I must be suffering from some kind of mental block. Yes, despair was setting in.

About three am I started to get a pain in my abdomen and it was growing more and more uncomfortable. After yet another one of my many visits to the bathroom I was returning to my bed and found it most difficult to climb into my bed. My abdomen pain was getting worse, and I was literally gasping as I tried to get into bed.

Fortunately, my night nurse was at that moment passing by and he came over to assist me. He was a big guy, built like an All Black prop and he easily lifted me up and tucked me into bed. He noticed my wincing expression as my pain persisted and pressed my abdomen that produced a yelp of pain from me. He fetched a machine and performed tummy scan on me and showed I had several litres of fluid in my abdomen. "My god" he exclaimed, "You are dangerously bloated! I am going to flush you out immediately."

With that he gathered together an array of instruments, tubes and basins etc and proceeded to insert a tube up my uthera. He then turned on a valve and the fluids literally spurted from my body into the basin. I can tell you the relief was miraculous. I sobbed as the release took place. After a spell of several minutes as I just lay there recovering, my saviour advised me that he would next insert a new catheter and I was introduced to My Catheter No 10.

You may have noticed I called my night nurse 'my saviour'. In keeping with my policy of no names no pack drill I have decided to refer to this man as "my saviour" because I believe that what he did next probably saved my life! He asked me to get out of bed, which he would then remake for me so I could be more comfortable and get some sleep. So I did as requested and sat on the chair while he remade my bed. It was now 4 am and had been a long night.

When the bed was ready I got to my feet to get back into it and had a dizzy spell and nearly fell over. Luckily my saviour caught me and physically lifted me back into bed. I must have almost fainted and in fact I was 'away with the fairies' as the saying goes. "Enough is enough," said my saviour, " I am going to summon the duty doctor to check you out".

A petite young Japanese lady doctor arrived within 10 minutes and went over my body with her stethoscope. My blood pressure was also checked and she said my heart was racing way above normal. She said she would organise a full ECG check in the morning and in the meantime prescribed some Panadol tablets to help get me off to sleep.

I didn't need much help, by now I was quite exhausted and I did manage a couple of hour's good sleep. When I woke up

I asked to see my saviour, but unfortunately he had finished his shift and had gone home. No doubt he needed some rest as well. What a man, what a fine example of fulfilling his duties, what a credit to his profession.

If I thought the night had been a drama filled adventure, the new day turned out to be even more adventurous. Not as dramatic perhaps, but nevertheless filled with so many incidents the new day deserves a separate chapter. My Catheter and I invite you to come along with us.

CHAPTER 9

OH WHAT A DAY.

After my unpleasant and at times frightening night experiences I was rather abruptly awoken when a couple of nurses trundled a heart monitoring machine into my room and proceeded to fit several small suction caps to various parts of my body. I think there were 16 of them. To these they attached lengths of wire cables which all lead into a multi plug which were hooked up to the monitor machine.

If I was a bit sleepy when they started—I was wide-awake now! They told me that following my dizzy spell during the night the doctor had ordered an ECG to be done and the results were to be relayed from my bedside machine to the main hospital computer so specialist heart staff could keep a watch on my progress during the day. An intravenous drip feed was plugged into the back of my hand and a bag of fluid was set up on a stand. When the nurses thought all was ready they switched me on. Nothing happened!

More nurses were called to my room, there was I surrounded by six nurses and tied to a couple of machines by 16 cables! The cables became the centre of attention as each one was checked that it had been hooked up correctly. A couple were found to be suspect and my chest hair was even shaved off and they were reattached. The machine was switched on again and this time it whirred into life.

A printout was produced and more fine-tuning was done. A phone message came through to the head nurse that nothing was being transmitted downstairs to the central computer monitoring station. A mild panic set in: every contact point was rechecked, there were by now eight nurses crowded round my bed seeking the reason for the problem. I overheard the youngest nurse, a Korean girl ask the charge nurse "Have you done this before?" The look the young nurse received from the charge nurse could have been interpreted in any language. I didn't help any when I started to laugh, but I was asking myself the same question.

Suddenly some bright spark came up with a suggestion that perhaps the port plug the Heart Monitor was plugged into was out of order. It was! The mild panic now became more urgent, what to do? The answer was simple; shift me to another room. Another exodus took place. My bed with me in it, the three machines I was plugged into and my personal belongings were all trundled out of the room and into another close by. Here I was set up again, machines, bed, drip-feeds my belongings, I was ready for business, but were the hospital staff? No they were not! The computer port in this room was out of order also! Have you ever laughed with tears in your eyes? I have.

You may find this hard to believe, but another shift took place! Yes, the whole caboodle lock stock and barrel was shifted into yet a third room! I must say this room was in the five star class. Down one wall it was sheer glass, a window with a great view out over the Waitemata Harbour. What's more the computer port worked because a message came through that the control room was receiving data loud and clear, I could even watch my heart rate on a Technicolor screen.

I have to tell you that my breakfast had been following me from room to room and by now it was 10.30 am. Breakfast was cold but I was damn hungry. There were just two nurses left tidying up for me and one of them trundled my breakfast trolley over the central part of my bed so I could sit up and eat it. You would not believe what happened next! I suddenly had an urgent need to pee! There I was sitting up in bed with my breakfast trolley positioned over my mid section and there was no bed bottle or basin to be seen. I couldn't push the trolley away from my upright sitting posture; it must have had a break on it.

After two days and a night trying desperately to produce a pee of quantity and quality I had wasted it—I had wet the bed! I was quite mortified and somewhat embarrassed. I had to buzz for the nurse and explain what had happened. As luck would have it the nurse who came to my help was the young Korean girl I mentioned previously, I half expected her to ask me if I had done this before! But she got me out of bed, changed my hospital dressing gown, seated me on a chair and even wheeled my breakfast trolley over to where I was sitting so I could finish breakfast while she remade my bed. Great!

The day so far was like a classic Marx Brothers movie, just when you think nothing more could possibly happen something did. In retrospect, I now see the funny side of all I am telling you, but if you had to re-enact it you couldn't do it. So to continue, at that moment I receive a visitor, my son Louis and he was most welcome. I described my previous night to him and the furore of the morning. He was most amused in a polite sort of way, and anyway being able to tell him was therapeutic in some way.

We were able to acquire a cup of coffee each from the mid morning tea and coffee trolley and talked on for a while until it was time for Louis to go. He stood up and made a sweeping gesture to shake hands with me and knocked my cup of coffee off the trolley straight into my lap! I jumped up out of my chair but I was drenched in coffee and standing in a puddle. I had pulled some of the computer wires off my back and I was the cause of alarm bells sounding from my computer and presumably down in the control room!

Louis is a quick thinker; he hurried out to the reception desk and told them his father had spilled his hot coffee over himself! It was nurses galore again. Louis didn't bother coming back to make sure I was ok, he just quietly left for home. The nurses made short work of tidying up and once again I was in a cosy bed and everything had been restored to normal. When my heart monitor came to life again it was sitting on a steady pulse rate of 60 and the medical people seemed pleased with that. In any case all the kafuffle I had been subjected to over the last few hours should have let them know I was sound of heart, I had to be didn't I?

By mid afternoon I had settled down. The drip feed was removed and I was able to unplug my heart monitor and have a shower. I still had 16 plugs stuck on by body but they were surplus to the hospital needs now. My heart was all ok. But my adventure was not over yet. Two nurses I hadn't seen before came to tell me the doctors required chest x-rays and they would wheel me down to the x-ray room.

The trip in the lift and down to the third floor was a fun trip. We laughed and joked and one of the nurses commented that she thought I was eying up the various nurses we passed on our travels. I told them that never in my life had I had my private parts prodded and handled by so many nubile young women who were probably well aware they were quite safe. We arrived at an x-ray room and had to wait outside until it became vacant.

The door opened and a cot containing a very young baby was wheeled out. It was too much; I broke into tears at the sad sight. I noticed both the nurses had tears in their eyes also. One remarked to me "That's why I can't work in the children's ward. While I was in the x-ray room I said some prayers for the child, you have probably surmised by now I am a softy at heart and at times somewhat prone to prayer.

Late in the afternoon the parade of doctors did their rounds and I was pleased to be told that I would be discharged the next day but with a catheter and I would receive regular checks by the District Nurses. The nurses and the Urology Clinic would be in touch frequently and any decisions made would be conveyed to me.

What a day it had been—oh what a day!

CHAPTER 10

A STEP FORWARD AND TWO BACKWARDS

My discharge from hospital following my operation was a relief to say the least; a male nurse attended to me and busied himself fitting a new catheter to me—number 10. I was quite excited about going home after five nights and six days after being shifted from pillar to post as it were. I really didn't' pay much attention to what the nurse was doing, I just wanted him to get the job done and let me go.

My wife picked me up and drove me home and I can tell you the intensity of my emotions about coming home were enough to bring tears to my eyes. It was only about an hour after my homecoming that I realised something was wrong with the way my catheter tubing had been arranged.

The tube from my uthera to the bag was too short and the bag itself was too small! The bag was fitted over my knee and when I had to bend my knee, pressure was put on the tube, which seemed to pull it out of my uthera. Just the act of sitting down or standing up applied pressure. It was quite painful at times and I spent a most uncomfortable and mainly sleepless night in bed.

Next morning I contacted the District Nurses office and explained the problem to them. They said they would send a nurse out shortly and about an hour later she duly arrived. She took one look at the way the male nurse had fitted No 10 catheter and removed the bag. She was going to extend the tube and fit a larger bag beneath my knee when she came up with a different idea.

She suggested simply fitting an on/off tap to the short catheter tube so whenever I had the urge to pee or to drain my bladder all I had to do was flick the tap from the off position into the on position and pass the fluid into a container. Brilliant! I thought the idea was a real step forward. I had become 'switched on' as it were. And I have to say it was decidedly comfortable, the tap although large fitted snugly between my thighs—it was like an extended penis!

It was a bright sunny day and my wife had decided to plant some new flowers in our entry garden. I was able to help her by passing her plants and generally tidying up after her by removing empty flower punnets and sweeping up. Over the next couple of hours I did feel the urge to pee, but when I readied myself for the big moment and was positioned over the container and then turned my tap on—you guessed it—nothing happened!

I couldn't believe it! I flicked the tap on and off many times, but to no avail. The same thing happened all the rest of the day and evening. I went to bed that night and I have say it was very comfortable laying in bed and being able to stretch out without all the tubes and bags getting in your way when you rolled over to get into a more comfortable position. For some reason I prefer to sleep on one side or the other, but sleeping on my back is to me most uncomfortable. Unfortunately sleeping on your back most suits wearing of catheters, sleeping on your side does not! You often get into tangles.

About two in the morning I woke up to recurring spasms of pain in my abdomen. The pain was occurring at about 10 minute intervals and the pain intensity was increasing. I started to writhe about and was gasping and moaning to the extent my wife said "That's enough, get up I'm taking you to the hospital!" So it was back to the Emergency Clinic about 4 am. During the drive in the pain spasms became quicker and more intense. I was in agony!

They didn't muck around at the hospital, it was into a room, a quick check of my heart and blood pressure and off with the offending tap and a major flush out of my bladder done. I can tell you the relief was instantaneous and tremendous. My doctor was a Russian fellow and he supervised the whole proceedings.

I was emptied out and allowed to just lie there making contented sighing noises, it really was a great feeling of relief, I had never experienced pain like it before. My Russian doctor said I was brought in just in time, my bladder could have ruptured and then I would have been in really big trouble.

Anyway, the doctor fitted No 11 catheter, this time I was able to show him the positioning I found most comfortable and he agreed with me. He went ahead and got me ready for my discharge and when he presented my discharge papers to me he pointed out a sentence that stated the tap that had been fitted to the catheter tube had been faulty, it didn't operate at all.

So in less than 24 hours I had experienced what I considered had been a major step forward and a major step backwards. I couldn't help feeling I was doomed, I was caught in the grip of My Catheter and it was hanging on for dear life, my experience that night convinced me it was my life it was hanging on for.

CHAPTER 11

NEW HOPE—HOPE DASHED.

I was at home and Catheter No 10 was doing its job well. I was passing fluid regularly and in reasonable quantities and I felt I was at last on the mend. My hopes were high; I even felt that My Catheter and I were at last working together.

I think it was on the Thursday morning, one week after my Russian doctor had taken care of the non-functioning tap problem that I received a phone call from a District Nurse to say she was calling on me within the hour to remove my Catheter! My hopes reached an all time high; I believed I was ready to return to normal. YipPEE!

The nurse arrived within the hour and had a look at my No 10 catheter and advised that the Doctors wanted it removed and then they wanted me to pass fluid into a container over the next four hours, which I had to measure and keep a record of. She would return in four hours time to examine the results and then make a decision whether to leave me catheter free or to insert a new one.

The Nurse's information was not quite what I had decided in my mind, the catheter removal was really a trial to determine if I could manage without it. If you will recall, I had been subjected to a similar trial a few days after No 1 catheter had been inflicted upon me for a similar trial and I had failed that at the time. But I was more confident this time.

The nurse left me with the advice to drink plenty of water to help flush my bladder.

Over the past three months I have received the water message countless number of times from all kinds of people. And what's more, I have diligently followed that advice. I am positive my bladder is always full, but it seems my bladder is reluctant to runneth over!

Anyway, the nurse left me to it and it was down to serious work. I can only describe my newfound release from a catheter as divine. I was able to stand there unencumbered by tubes and attached bags and pee! I honestly did as I had been instructed; I passed fluid into the container and measured it carefully. I was pleased with my performance and for the record here are my results.

In the three hours the trial lasted I drank two litres of water and a couple of cups of coffee. I was able to pass fluid roughly every half an hour. My first flow was only 2 ml, but from then on it increased from 52 ml and peaked at 105 ml a couple of times. My total was 660 ml. I was quite elated; I thought I had done really well. And I felt good as well; I felt the best I had been for a considerable time.

The nurse arrived back an hour sooner than expected telling me she was behind on her calls that day so she was saving time. She inspected the records I had kept and then told me she needed to do a tummy reading to check on the amount of fluid I was still holding. She produced a hand held battery powered recording device and proceeded to run it over my abdomen. She did this several times.

The nurse told me she thought the battery in her device could be flat as she was getting a different reading each time she tried! She didn't have a replacement battery in her bag or in her car, but in any case her results showed I was still holding too much fluid in my bladder and she would have to reinsert another catheter! I was devastated and pleaded with her, but she was adamant.

So it was on my back again while catheter No 11 was inserted. I was close to tears despite the nurses assurances that what was happening to me was quite common in cases where a prostate removal had been done! I protested that my prostate had not been removed, only reamed out. But she would have none of that and even produced a discharge document that she said plainly stated my prostate had been removed.

What with my failure to pass sufficient fluid, a faulty battery on her measuring device, and news that my prostate had been removed, my confidence had been shattered—my hope had been dashed. What to do now?

The first thing I did do was phone the District Nurses organisation and question the information about the record their visiting nurse had claimed showed my prostate had been removed. She advised me that was indeed the case and I would have a copy of the document in my letterbox the next morning.

The next thing I did was telephone the Green Lane Urology Clinic and explain my confusion about whether my prostate had been removed or not? After a few moments a member of the team that I was registered with came on the phone and assured me that the prostate definitely had not been removed. I was asked why would a benign prostate be removed? At least that was good information!

Anyway, what with all the goings on such as tests, results, operation reports and several phone calls, the next development was that I received a phone call from the Green Lane Urology Clinic to attend an appointment the following week with the Surgeon who had operated on me for a check up. My Catheter and I remained bound together.

CHAPTER 12

THE INS AND OUTS OF THE MATTER

The time for my appointment at the Green Lane Urology Clinic duly arrived and I turned up 30 minutes early to ensure a place in the pecking order. I only had a 10-minute wait when my doctor's nurse came and fetched me and ushered me into a small operating room. She explained that my surgeon was going to inspect my internal prostate wound with a microscopic camera and to do that my catheter would need to be removed.

So it was off with my pants and underwear and onto the cot. The nurse deftly removed the catheter, sterilised my exposed parts and had me laid out ready for the inspection. In came my surgeon and he had a cursory look at my parts and outlined what was about to happen to me.

The problem had risen due to my prostate been greatly oversized. In my original operation a large portion of the prostate had been reamed out via a flexible tube inserted through my uthera. The operating process had taken some time and as a result I was left with quite a large wound.

Residual prostate tissue was left inside me and it was most certainly remnants of this residual matter that had caused the few times my catheter had blocked which was unfortunate but quite common after the type of operation he had performed.

With that he inserted his camera tube up my uthera and started to look about. Do you know I could actually watch proceedings happening inside me on a colour computer screen! There was hardly any pain involved, and the surgeon was even able to show me small portions of residual matter floating about in my bladder. It was amazing and somewhat unreal.

The internal examination came to an end and the next step was the insertion of My Catheter No 12. To be honest I was quite relieved that this ordeal was over, it is interesting yes, but the process does involve a degree of tension and stress. The surgeon advised me that thanks to his inspection he had found that a small clean up operation would be required and he was booking me into Hospital for this to be done on July 29th.

He told me not to worry, it was a straightforward cleanup operation and he was sure I would be able to resume a normal lifestyle afterwards. He did remind me that he had mentioned the possible need for a further operation after he had performed the first one, which I did recall. With that he shook my hand and said he would see me on the 29th and left.

I thought my clinic visit was over, but not so. The nurse then told me she needed to up date the medical records they held for me. So I was taken through the whole gambit yet again; my height, my weight, blood pressure, blood sugar, heart, and so forth. I think that over the three months this missal has covered to date this routine must have now happened about 10 times!

I left the clinic quite pleased with what had happened. The procedures used and the explanations given all seemed perfectly logical and I had already started resigning myself to having my No 12 catheter for another month or so. But alas, it was not to be, the Malediction that existed between My Catheter and I descended on me yet again.

It was only two days after my Clinic visit that I found the damn catheter No 12 had become blocked again! It was Saturday night about 10 pm and my discomfort was growing with shooting pains happening in my abdomen. My dear wife was by now used to what was needed—back to the AHB Emergency Clinic. We had no alternative; the Urology Clinic at Green Lane did not operate after hours.

Because no fluid was being discharged through my catheter into the attached bag, the fluid forces itself through the uthera and out the penis with great force. This happened to me twice that evening and I can tell you the experience is most distressing. If you are not quick enough everything is wet, it is embarrassing and a major clean up is necessary.

At the AHB I was taken to a room where a nurse helped me disrobe and established me on the bed. She removed the catheter bag leaving only the tube. She quickly and efficiently pumped 25 ml of fluid into me to enable a flushing out of my bladder. Nothing happened! A young doctor from Taiwan came into the room and quickly organised a drip system into my body and also an intravenous drip feeder through the back of my hand. A large catheter bag was reattached to the tube and fluid started to flow.

My Taiwanese doctor revisited me and told me I would be staying overnight, so I phoned my wife with the news and she told me I was in the best place and she would go to bed herself as she now didn't have to pick me up. Both my initial nurse and doctor had finished their shift and were duly replaced by a new duo.

The new nurse came in and inspected my fluid flow into the bag. She told me she would be back in a few minutes with the doctor as she felt he would want to have an inspection himself. I was somewhat alarmed about her comments, but the new doctor arrived and lo and behold was the Russian doctor who had attended me and changed my catheter on my previous visit. He too closely inspected the catheter bag.

He showed me the bag and commented about the large amount of residual matter that had been flushed out. He asked me if I might have an idea why there was such a discharge. Then the penny dropped! I told him about my visit to Green lane less than two days ago and the internal inspection my surgeon had made. I recalled the surgeon telling me he had stirred things up a bit inside me and blockages might happen.

My Russian doctor agreed that the reason was valid and that the prime blockage had been successfully cleaned out. He then had all the flushing tubes disconnected and told me he was going to insert a new catheter and I could go home! Once again an emotive euphoria took over my thinking. I was relieved of my stress because I had been advised a new blockage might happen and it had. Better still the problem had been fixed. My Catheter and I would carry on the journey; I did ask myself if catheter No 13 might have some significance in future progress?

It was 2 am when I was discharged and caught a taxi home. I arrived about 15 minutes past two am and walked up to my front door. I knocked quietly so as not to disturb family, but there was no activity. I then gently called my wife's name, but still no action. Then I had a brainwave, I made a cat call! A meow believe it or not, imitating our cat calling to get in! There was an instant response with my wife traipsing down the corridor half asleep to let me in. She told me she knew it wasn't the cat because it was asleep on the bed beside her. Believe me, the meow call worked, that's my story and I am sticking to it.

CHAPTER 13

LET'S GO ON WITH THE SHOW.

In the previous chapter I described how I had become acquainted with My Catheter No 13 and I expressed the hope that number 13 might prove a lucky number for me. Procedures were now moving ahead at a fast rate and I had already been told that a second operation would be done on the 29th July. But before the actual operation date arrived there was another procedure I had to undergo before the main show could start, I had to revisit the Urology Clinic at Green Lane for another "Pre Op" examination.

Now I have previously mentioned my first Pre-Admission Clinic, but this time I want to let you know just what happens during the three or four hours this clinic takes. I have also previously made comment on the multi mixture of various nationalities of the medical staff I have been attended to during the several months this account has taken to unfold so far. 20 different doctors, and probably double that number of male and female nursing staff must have attended me to. Believe it or not, only one doctor and about 10 nurses were kiwis!

I want to use this chapter to illustrate the multi national factor I have experienced.

I arrived at the Clinic at 9 am and registered myself at the reception desk. I was told to take a seat until my name was called. About 15 minutes later I was called back to the desk and handed a sheet of paper and told to report to the Cardiology Department up on the next floor, which I did. Again I was told to take a seat until my name was called.

After a 15 minute wait I was called and ushered into a small room where I had to remove my upper clothing and lie down on a cot where several plugs were attached to various parts of my torso and an ECG examination was conducted and a print out of the results was produced by a machine which my examiner carefully scrutinised before handing me the print out which he told me was a good result; and instructed me to take it back to the downstairs reception. The ECG examiner was from Samoa.

Once again I was asked to take a seat until my name was called. Another 15 minutes lapsed before the call came. This time a nurse who explained to me that it was her job to take me to the various medical staff who would be involved in one way or another in my forthcoming operation for me to meet. The nurse was from Zimbabwe and a bit hard to understand.

Before delivering me to the medical people I would be meeting, the Zimbabwe nurse weighed me, measured my height, recorded my temperature and took my blood pressure. I have lost count of the number of times these procedures have taken place over the past few months, but I assume that it is easier to make new recordings that look up past records.

My first meeting was with the House Surgeon whom was from Iran. He did have all the records of my previous operation and advised me he would be assisting my surgeon, who by the way is from England, at my forthcoming operation. He explained to me that a tidy up operation was fairly normal after the type of operation I had previously experienced. In fact, he told me, about 40% of such operations required a follow up, so I shouldn't worry too much about it. He also said that about 20% of the follow up operations still required a period of flushing out of the bladder and it could take up to a year before things were back to normal!

By now you know how much I like delving into statistics, so let's do it again. If 40 people in 100 require a follow up operation, and 8 of those still need attention I don't know if I can prevent myself worrying about it, it's there in your mind isn't it? Will My Catheter NO 13 prove to be lucky for me?

My next visit was to the Anaesthetist, an Englishman, who spent considerable time discussing with me his role in the forthcoming operation. He was particularly interested in my previous experience. Believe it or not all I could tell him was that I could not recall much at all about it. I was wheeled into the operating theatre, put to sleep and woke up four hours later being wheeled into my ward—room. I could honestly say there was no pain experience whatsoever. I told him I would like the same again.

It was explained carefully that a final decision on my anaesthetic method would be made on the day as circumstances would need to be considered first. I have to say that I consider these medical specialists deserve respect and admiration; they do a great job, before—during—and after their administrations.

So next my Zimbabwean nurse delivered me to a doctor who was Malaysian. He discussed my medical list, all the pills I take to keep my functions in tune. I actually take eight pills a day faithfully and they do seem to produce good results. So after determining why I took these prescribed pills I was assured by the doctor that I should continue with the medication and have regular check ups with my personal doctor.

Then it was off to meet the Pre Op Consultant, also Iranian whom I had met before on my first Pre Op visit. Once again she discussed all the various procedures I would have to follow to gain admission to the Hospital on admission day. These procedures range from confirming you will be arriving and the Hospital will tell you what time they want you to report. You are given a fully itemised list of what you must do and what you need to bring with you. The documentation the Consultant hands you is very concise and a great help.

The Consultant then took me to the Blood Testing Laboratory where a very efficient nurse extracted three tubes of blood from me. To complete my nationality roster, this nurse was a Kiwi.

So there you are, a description of what the Pre—Op Clinic is all about and a list that reveals that of the seven people who attended to me only one was a kiwi. I happen to think it is remarkable how much our Medical System depends on overseas recruitment for their staff, and I can testify on what a great job they all do.

By the way, there was an offshoot to my Pre Op visit that day; I also had to visit the Retinal Clinic on the first floor in the same building. This was my bi-annual vision testing to check out my eyesight. During this visit you are attended by two people, the first was a lady who puts the drops into your eyes, she was from China and the second was the man who does the actual photography work. He was from South Africa. Just thought you might be interested in that extra information. By the way my tests were all ok. I don't suppose there is a connection there with My Catheter 13!

Roll on July 29th, I am prepared, let the show begin!

CHAPTER 14

ONCE MORE INTO THE FRAY!

August the 29th, a Friday came along and once more my Catheter and I had to turn up at the Hospital for the resumption with our "Battle of the Prostate". We turned up at the pre appointed time of 11.30 am and reported to the admittance counter.

We (My catheter and I) were conducted to a waiting room where a nurse dosed me with a couple of Panadol tablets, did a blood sugar test, took all my clothes off me and fitted me with a back the front dressing gown. Another nurse fitted me with special Medic-Stockings and escorted me back to the waiting room. I was I suppose dressed and ready for battle. I noticed seven wheeled beds lined up in the passage next to the waiting room and as I waited I counted seven other combatants dressed in similar garb to me.

"Bring it on" I thought to myself, I am ready, yes "Once more into the fray!" But before battle commenced there was one more a session with my Anaesthetist I had to go through. It was explained to me that I would be put to sleep using the same method as my first operation five weeks previously. This was merely a 'clean up operation' and it was not expected to carry any unseen problems with it.

In fact my anaesthetist seemed more interested in the origin of my surname and when I explained it was Italian he started speaking in Italian to me! I was delivered into the operating theatre at 12.45 pm where several nurses started procedures and the very last thing I remember is the smiling face of my anaesthetist beaming down at me and him saying 'Bourn Giorno Giovanni Francesco Battista!"

I awoke in the Ward where I had a single bedroom and it had a window view and a private shower and toilet. A quick inspection revealed I now had a new catheter. I was sorry I had missed the opportunity to officially farewell Catheter 13 as it had performed well for the two weeks we had been together.

Let me tell you that My Catheter No 14 made a somewhat ignominious start to our relationship! It had been set in place about 3.13 pm and by 6.15 pm it had become blocked by residual matter from my operation! All I could say to myself was "here I go again!" I had been told that these blockages were a common happening after my type of operation and two nurses soon had the blockage flushed away and things were operating smoothly.

My Surgeon paid a visit that afternoon and told me he was very pleased how it had all gone according to expectations. He reassured me that blockages were expected and may happen again, but eventually he expected me to be rid of my catheter and be able to pee normally. All I could say was YipPEE—WhooPEE—and HapPEE! He did warn me though that if the current operation did not fully produce the expected results, in future I might have to insert a Catheter myself on a daily basis to relieve bladder pressure!

I had a bastard of a night. The male nurse turned out to be more of a nuisance that a help. He was the same guy who attended me prior to my discharge from my first operation. You may recall he stuffed up the fitting of my catheter No 10 and it was the District Nurse who came to the rescue although her good intentions led me having to report to the Emergency Clinic at the hospital the next day.

Excuse the digression, and now back to my dissatisfaction with the male night nurse. He came into my room every few minutes flashing his flashlight all round the place including into my eyes. He performed his specific duties ok, like fiddling around with my drip feed bottles, my catheter flushing bottles; he emptied the catheter bags frequently.

Then about half way through the night he decided I needed to re-connected with the oxygen supply tubes—one through each nostril. He fiddled about refitting the tubes and somehow I ended up with a tube wrapped around each ear and then both tubes wrapped around my throat under my chin.

The oxygen fitting was damned uncomfortable and most irritating. On his next visit I told him it was worrying me and told him I didn't think I needed it. I asked him politely if he would remove it, but he replied that he did think I needed it and refused to take it off. So the rest of the night went sleepless. When the new staff came on duty in the morning the first thing the new nurse asked what I was doing with the oxygen tubes wrapped around my head and removed them! An angel had rescued me.

A male nurse from Ethiopia helped me to shower early that morning and after breakfast I must say that despite the bad night I did feel quite a new man. Things improved greatly when my surgeon accompanied by his usual retinue of young doctors and again expressed his satisfaction over my progress. He ordered My Catheter No 14 be removed and I had pee naturally into a jug and have the nurses measure discharge.

Oh Bliss, delightful bliss. Right from the start I passed fluid, quite bloody yes, but also regular and in good quantities. There was no pain involved and I knew when it was time to go. And it got better and better as the day went on. I was able to walk around quite easily and I made sure I drank water copiously as I had been instructed. The more water I drank the clearer my discharges became.

When my surgeon made his late afternoon visit he was most pleased and said things were on track as he had hoped. He said he was confident he would discharge me the next day.

I then pleaded with him to let me go home for the evening as I had purchased a new 55 inch HD TV and had yet to see a top Rugby game on it. The All Blacks were playing the Springboks that night and that was one of the main reasons I had purchased the set.

He thought about my somewhat impassioned plea and to my joy agreed to me having "Leave of Absence" for the night as long as I undertook to be back in Hospital by 7.30 am the next morning. He made a condition that I was refitted with another catheter for my overnight visit. So catheter No 15 was quickly fitted and as luck had it, my daughter had just come to visit me and was able to drive me home.

When we arrived at home I realised I didn't have a door key and my wife wasn't home. Then I remembered my next-door neighbour had a spare key just in case of emergencies like this and my daughter ran up the drive to fetch the key. On her return she preceded me to unlock the door and I went to ascend the three steps onto the front porch. Would you believe I tripped on the bottom step? I actually fell up the steps! I twisted my left ankle and I burst open the catheter bag on my right leg.

I was in a painful mess. My Catheter and I had parted company only after an hour or so in each other's company. I was able to partially retrieve the situation with my daughters help; she is a full time nurse at Waitakere Hospital. I was able to clean up the bloodied mess before my wife arrived home. I was also able to rig up a new catheter bag to contain any discharge and decided I would put up with the ankle pain and watch the big game despite the ankle pain.

I have to be honest and tell you that on my wife's return home she berated my idea to come home just because of a damned rugby game! "Bloody ridiculous" she told me over and over, and in fact she still repeats that opinion to this day. I sat through the game in some discomfort and as soon as it was over I went to bed.

Yet again sleep was difficult and I discovered my makeshift catheter bag was leaking. At 3 am I decided I had better get back to hospital and phoned for a taxi as I felt the time was not right to ask my wife to drive me. I arrived back at the hospital and I must say the night staffs was quite surprised to see me at that hour of the morning. I was delighted to find the night nurse on duty was none other than my saviour you have already met in Chapter 8.

I was put back into my original bed and not long after by the night doctor—from Egypt would you believe? After inspecting my new catheter bag he spent considerable time examining my ankle. He gently twisted and turned it, bent it backwards and then forwards and then made me walk forwards and backwards as he observed my walking ability. He then ordered me back to bed and told me he would send me for an x-ray in the morning.

I can say I slept really well and was woken up for breakfast. Immediately after finishing my morning meal I was again visited by my surgeon and his train of young doctors. He had been told about my tripping accident and my early return to hospital. He ordered the removal of Catheter 15 and a resumption of measuring my discharges during the day. I can report that everything went well and I was told I would need to stay yet another night as a precaution resulting from my fall.

At 7.30 pm that day I was suddenly shifted from my top class bedroom into another room to share with three guys. One poor guy had just come out of a gall stone operation and was in great pain and moaned considerably. The second guy also had urology problems and he also groaned quite a bit. Perhaps I should describe his murmurings as moaning rather than groaning. You know—the complaining type of moaning rather than pain caused groaning, in between moans he spent considerable time on a cell phone. The last guy simply slept most of the time.

As for me I was catheter free and unencumbered by any of the tubes and bags I had lived with over the previous months. I was discharging very well; I was able to walk about, shave, shower and shampoo and made time to call on my roommates to discuss our problems. I was able to discern that I was better off physically and probably mentally than any one of them. I must tell you that during most of the night we had a marvellous night nurse who tended to each of us with magnificent dedication. She administered her duties with tireless energy and a degree of cheerfulness that boosted our morale. We each kept telling each other just how wonderful this woman was.

The next morning the Doctors daily visit happened again and I was delighted to have my discharge later in the day confirmed. I was then taken away for my ankle x-rays which were later confirmed as all ok by a physio—therapist. My performances had met the doctor's standards and I could go home!

Somewhere in this chapter I remarked YipPEE—WhooPEE—and HapPEE! And those exclamations are intended as a reflection on my jubilant feelings. Of course the emphasis is on PEE! That is what it is all about. But the story of My Catheter and I is not quite over yet. Six weeks after my discharge I am required to visit my Surgeon for a final check-up. That is when the final chapter will be written. That is when I will bid my farewell to my Catheter. I can't wait.

www.ingramcontent.com/pod-product-compliance
Lightning Source LLC
Chambersburg PA
CBHW022126170526
45157CB00004B/1772